Unsere gemeinsame Zeit

Impressum:
Manuela Vogt
Am Wohld 24
24244 Felm
E-Mail: vergiss-mein-nicht@gmx.net

www.ingramcontent.com/pod-product-compliance
Lightning Source LLC
Chambersburg PA
CBHW060854220526
45466CB00003B/1365